The
EDEN
DIET

WORKBOOK

You Can **Eat** Treats,
Enjoy Your Food,
and **Lose** Weight

By

Rita Hancock, MD

The EDEN DIET

WORKBOOK

This book belongs to:

_____

The Eden Diet Workbook
Copyright 2008 by Personalized Fitness Products, LLC;
Oklahoma City, Oklahoma, USA

" 'The Eden Diet Workbook' is an independent publication and is not affiliated with, sponsored by, or endorsed by Eden Foods, Inc."

ISBN 978-0-9820341-1-8

TABLE OF *Contents*

Introduction

WHAT IF YOU could eat whatever you wanted and still lose weight? And what if you could draw closer to the Lord and experience the fruit of the Spirit—peace, joy, love, and hope—in the process?

You can pinch yourself if you want to, but, I promise you're not dreaming. You're reading about a doctor-proven, patient-tested, Christ-centered weight control plan called the Eden Diet. It involves waiting until you're physically hungry and then eating smaller portions—of your favorite foods. The Eden Diet also involves eating with thankfulness and appreciation to God rather than with guilt and shame.

Perhaps I'm telling you what you already know. You were supposed to have read the main Eden Diet book in its entirety before starting this workbook.

If you didn't finish reading the main book, please go back and do so now. I'd like you to have a broad overview of the plan before you start the workbook exercises.

In the main book, I talk about how to attune to your hunger pangs, how to trim down portion sizes, and how to recognize and combat the emotions, mindless habits, and advertising messages that lead you to eat when you aren't actually hungry.

In the workbook, I expand on these principles and help you put what you learned into practice. In addition, I give you specific tools to help you combat urges to overeat at restaurants, buffets, and other food-related social events.

You may proceed through this workbook on your own or as part of a support group. Either way, I want you to pray about and meditate on the questions before you answer them. Don't think of the exercises as being chores on your "to do" list, and don't rush. The exercises are an opportunity for you to receive revelation knowledge from God and deeper emotional healing.

Even if it causes you to feel uncomfortable, try to answer the workbook questions honestly. But, don't feel obligated to share your answers in the support group meetings if you don't want to. If you say too much, the other members of the group might find out that you're not normal, like they are.

Okay, I hope you know I'm kidding. The truth is your crazy thoughts about food and eating are probably no crazier than anyone else's (especially if you're all females at the meeting), so don't be afraid to share. It's liberating.

Once you complete the workbook, you may cycle through it again as many times as you like. Often, you'll gain deeper insights on your second and third times through the material. If you run out of room in the workbook in which to journal or answer questions, start a separate journal to continue recording your insights.

If you join a support group that's already in progress, you might have to start working on exercises in the middle of the book rather than at the beginning. That's okay. You can start at any point in the workbook because each chapter covers a different topic. Just leave the earlier sections of the workbook unfinished and cycle through them later.

Toward the end of the workbook, you will find a food diary. It's to be used only by those who are not losing weight as quickly as expected. A food diary can help you discover if "mindless" eating is blocking your weight loss. But, the burden of having to keep a food diary can also keep you fixated on food and eating! So, use the diary only temporarily. Just long enough to figure out why you're not losing weight.

Finally, throughout the workbook, I encourage you to listen to the audio CDs entitled "Godly Affirmations for Weight Loss," which are available at this time ONLY through www.TheEdenDiet.com (and soon through iTunes). You may listen to the audio recordings at home or at the end of workshop meetings to support and reinforce healthier eating habits.

Please understand that the CDs are not "Eden Diet books on tape." Rather, they are relaxing, twenty to twenty-five minute fantasy exercises that reinforce and complement the material in the main book. They are like mini-mental-vacations that help you to de-stress so you feel less inclined to stress-eat.

For example, in the audio recording, "A Walk on the Beach," I ask you to fantasize that you're walking on the beach with the Lord. Meanwhile, I speak soothing, messages of His mercy and love to defuse the emotions that might otherwise trigger you to eat. All of this is set against relaxing background sounds of ocean waves and seagulls.

At the time of this printing, four different relaxation CDs are available. In addition to the beach CD, check out "A Walk in the Forest," which deals with learning to enjoy exercise, a "A Picnic at the Lake," which deals with learning how to eat properly at social events that center on food, and "A Battle With the Flesh," which deals with controlling your cravings.

At least two more CDs are planned for release in 2010, including one tentatively entitled, "Forgiveness Makes You Skinny," and another called "Letting Go of Strife."

To round out your Eden Diet experience, sign up for my free Blog articles and Eden Diet newsletter. The newsletter is published once-a-month-only (with no junk email in between) and is safe-subscribe, meaning we do not share your email address. The newsletter periodically includes articles by me and/or interviews with my weight control expert colleagues. To sign up for the newsletter, click on the relevant sign-up button at the bottom of the home page of www.TheEdenDiet.com.

To become an Eden Diet blog follower, click the "Blog" button on the home page of www.TheEdenDiet.com, and then click on the "Follow" button. That automatically connects you with my most recent blog articles.

On the Web site, you can also find out about additional study material as it becomes available, including a couple books that are still rolling around in my head, *The Eden Diet For Kids and Teens* and *The Eden Diet Emotional Healing Handbook*. I'll let you know as soon as they make it onto paper.

Now, let's get busy and find you some Eden Diet weight loss joy!

How to *Start* and *Run* an Eden Diet Support Group

A. **Who May Start a Group:** Workshops may be started by interested individuals or groups. The *Group Founder* (the one who initiates group formation) should become thoroughly familiar with the detailed meeting agenda that is provided in the next section, as he or she will likely be the one arranging for and running the first few meetings.

B. **Leadership:** At the first meeting, members should prayerfully consider who will be *group leaders*. There should be at least two, so that if one leader misses a meeting, the other may facilitate. The *group founder* may continue as a *group leader*. The leaders may alternate weeks if desired and should coordinate their schedules so that at least one is present at each meeting.

C. **Chain of Communication:** A *Group Secretary* should also be designated at that first meeting. The Group Secretary should collect members' and visitors' contact information, send out e-mail and/or telephone reminders about meetings, and send follow-up notes to visitors to facilitate answering their questions after they attend. In addition, non-officer members should collect each others' contact info (a template is provided in the back of the workbook). **Pre-meeting reminder emails** from the secretary are extremely important to keep the group's enthusiasm and attendance high. These notes help members to feel connected and remain informed even when they cannot attend. They should be sent out two to three days before each meeting. **Post-meeting summaries** from the secretary are equally important. They should include encouraging quotations from the book, short, written summaries of material covered in the prior meeting, workbook assignments for the next meeting, and the date, time, and location of the next meeting. However, post-meeting summaries should NOT include personal information about individual members without their permission.

D. **Prerequisites:** It is strongly recommended that each member read through *The Eden Diet* parent book in its entirety during the seven-day challenge before starting on the workbook and before attending the meetings.

E. **Registration:** New Eden Diet support groups are to register at www.TheEdenDiet.com. Please indicate if your group is open to new members.

F. **Group Size:** The recommended number of members per group meeting is six to ten, but as few as two can start a group. Groups may split if attendance is consistently too high for the group to stay focused.

G. **Age Requirements:** Because of its references to sexuality as it relates to body weight, the Eden Diet is geared toward adults, eighteen years of age and older. Exceptions may be made with parental consent and the cooperation of the members to adapt the meeting content accordingly.

H. **Frequency of Meetings.** The recommended frequency of meetings is every other week.

I. **Duration of Meetings.** The recommended duration is no longer than ninety minutes. That should allow time for review of the questions and playing of the audio relaxation recordings.

J. **Attendance.** Members should take attendance seriously — as a commitment to the other members in the group. After all, their inclusion into the group may have meant that others were excluded.

K. **Midstream Addition of New Members.** You should be able to join a group at any point and not feel lost. There are two reasons why. First, the sections of the workbook don't necessarily build on each other. Second, you are supposed to read *The Eden Diet* in its entirety (in the seven-day challenge) before joining the group. Thus, no concept in the workbook will be completely new to you. That flexibility also allows you to stay in the group and cycle through the program as many times as you like.

L. **Encourage diversity in the group.** Expect members of all shapes and sizes, male or female, from the late teens to the senior years, some with eating disorders and others with only a few minor bad habits they'd like to shake. The group may also welcome family members of those with such issues. No matter how different we may seem in terms of our appearance, we are all on the same journey.

M. **Report Your Progress.** Eden Diet participants are encouraged to report their weight loss successes, praise reports, frustrations, and concerns, as well as before and after photos to www.TheEdenDiet.com. Just click on the "Q&A" or "Contact Us" buttons at the top of the home page and submit your information. Indicate if you would like to submit before and after photos for publication on the Web site, and you will be contacted with further instructions.

Agenda for Eden Diet Meetings

1. **Opening Prayer.** (Everyone reads aloud)

PRAYER OF COMMITMENT

"Heavenly Father, please help me to uphold my commitment to this program. Transform my thinking about food at a pace that is right for me so that I make choices that are consistent with weight loss. Help me to eat only small amounts of food and only when I am actually hungry, and help me find ways to resist the urge to eat when I am not hungry. Encourage me when I am down and help me be honest with myself when it is difficult. Help me to forgive myself and others for past indiscretions that led to my weight gain. And help me to feel comfortable and satisfied in the resultant body shape and size that You set for me. Thank You, Father. Amen."

2. **Greetings/Business.**

- Introduce new members or guests *and record their contact information.* (It is especially important for the group leaders and secretary to collect this information.)

- If not already done, elect at least two *group leaders* and one group secretary to send out e-mail and telephone reminders about meetings.

- In case new members have not yet read the book, explain the basic concept of the book in a few sentences. Tell them: "*The Eden Diet* is about eating according to internal cues—hunger pangs—rather than external rules about what food to eat and at what time. It's also about eating smaller portions and turning to God in prayer for help to avoid temptation."

- Explain the group format to new members (they should complete the workbook questions before the meeting, and they should contemplate the questions prayerfully).

- Explain the meeting schedule, location, dates, and times, and discuss whether or not child care will be available.

- Other members are encouraged to collect contact information for each other so that they may communicate and encourage each other in between meetings. There is a template to record this information in the back of the workbook.

- The secretary should add new members' names to the e-mail roster to ensure that all members receive information updates when appropriate.

- Review meeting rules (see page 13)

3. **Share Eden Diet Experiences from the previous two weeks** (allow twenty minutes).

   - Members who are willing may share questions, difficulties, and frustrations about the prior two-week period.

   - Brainstorm solutions and give support, always focusing on the positive.

   - Share praise reports, accomplishments, and behavioral goals that have been met.

4. **Review Portions of the Workbook** (allow thirty minutes). The Group Leader will direct members to read questions from the workbook to open those points up for group discussion. Nobody should feel pressured to share their responses.

5. **Relaxation Exercise** (allow thirty minutes). Take a ten-minute break before- hand to allow members to use the restroom, loosen tight clothing, turn off cell phones, post a "Please be quiet" sign on the door, check the area for non-members who might be noisy and ask them to move, etc. Once you have ensured that the environment is conducive to relaxation, you may play one of the "Godly Affirmations for Weight Loss" CDs, which are available for purchase on www.TheEdenDiet.com.

6. **Establish date, time, and location for the next meeting.**

7. **Assign which section or questions are to be answered from the workbook prior to the next meeting.**

8. **Stand up, join hands in a circle, and pray an ad lib closing prayer that is inspired by the meeting.** Pray for each other, for the success of the group and the program, and for any other needs the group members have.

9. **As you finish praying, take note of who is standing to your right.** That is the person you will pray for during the next two weeks. Contact that person during the intervening two weeks, and support and encourage them.

Rules for Eden Diet Meetings

1. **Embrace diversity in the group.** Welcome members of any size and shape, and welcome family members of interested individuals. Don't assume a person's food-related problems are smaller because their body is smaller. You can be in bondage at any weight.

2. **Don't dominate the floor.** In any group setting, one or more members may be more vocal or dominant than the others, and that could be counterproductive for the group as a whole. It is important to allow equal time for each member who wants to share. Please keep comments brief.

3. **Acceptable topics of discussion at the meetings:** Avoid topics of conversation that glorify or exalt food. Do not share diet recipes, and do not give each other diet tips. Instead, focus on God and how He can help you identify and change your self-destructive attitudes and behaviors about food. Remember, Jesus is Lord and the food is not.

4. **Don't propagate dogma and don't be judgmental.** Don't advise other group members on what, when, why, or how much they should eat for weight loss, and don't harp on them to "eat healthy." The group's focus should be on learning to eat according to internal cues, eating smaller portions, and glorifying God. Healthier eating will most likely occur naturally and secondarily over time, as members break free from bondage to food.

PART *One*

a new *paradigm* for weight loss

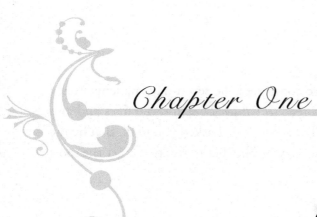

Chapter One

Overview of
The EDEN DIET

Begin the exercise in this chapter with the following prayer:

"Heavenly Father, clear my mind of dieting and nutrition dogma that confuses and misleads me and causes me to gain weight. Fill my mind with truth. Help me to understand the best way to lose weight. Thank You for Your endless mercy and grace. Amen."

In the space below record your insights after reading chapter 1 in *The Eden Diet*:

_____

_____

_____

_____

_____

_____

_____

_____

_____

_____

CHAPTER SUMMARY

If you are reading this workbook, then I assume you have completed the seven-day challenge that I outlined in *The Eden Diet*. The challenge required you to read *The Eden Diet* in seven days and also to begin to pay closer attention to your hunger signals and portion sizes. I asked you to do that before starting the exercises in this book. You need the broad overview of the diet to be able to get the most out of your first thirty days.

EXERCISE 1.1
THE SEVEN-DAY CHALLENGE

EXERCISE 1.1-A

In the space below, record your experience on the seven-day challenge. What were your insights, your successes, and your failures or frustrations?

_____

_____

_____

_____

EXERCISE 1.1-B

At this point, what obstacles do you foresee to succeeding on the Eden Diet?

_____

_____

_____

_____

EXERCISE 1.1-C

Pray and meditate on ways to overcome those obstacles.

_____

_____

_____

_____

EXERCISE 1.1-D

"The Old Me." In the space below, attach a current picture of yourself. Under, it, write "The Old Me." Remember, God loves you just the way you are right now, but He also loves you too much to leave you that way.

EXERCISE 1.1-E

"The New Me I Am Becoming." God speaks of things to come as though they already exist. Now, it's time for you to do the same. In the space below, affix a photo of a person who has a similar body shape to yours, only smaller. It may be a photo of you before you gained unwanted weight or a photo of someone else who is thinner and has similar proportions. In the space below the picture, write "The New Me." *Study this picture intently. Memorize it. This is the body you will visualize yourself in as you listen to the Godly Affirmations for Weight Loss CDs.*

EXERCISE 1.1-F

Eating habits. List ten changes in your eating habits that will help you eat less and become the leaner, stronger you that is shown in the second picture. You don't have to make all of the changes right now. Feel free to review the main book for ideas, if necessary.

1. _____
   _____

2. _____
   _____

3. _____
   _____

4. _____
   _____

5. _____
   _____

6. _____
   _____

7. _____
   _____

8. _____
   _____

9. _____
   _____

10. _____
    _____

EXERCISE 1.1-G

Exercise habits. List five changes in your exercise habits that will help you become the leaner, stronger you that is shown in the second picture.

1. _____
   _____

2. _____
   _____

3. _____
   _____

4. _____
   _____

5. _____
   _____

EXERCISE 1.1-H

Prayer habits. List five changes in your prayer and meditation habits that will help you to become the leaner, stronger you shown in the second picture.

1. _____
   _____

2. _____
   _____

3. _____
   _____

4. _____
   _____

5. _____
   _____

EXERCISE 1.1-I

Decrease triggers for overeating. List five changes in your lifestyle that could help to decrease your triggers for overeating. For example, if stress leads you to eat, identify the cause of the stress (e.g. finances, over-commitment of time, etc.), and, if possible, reduce or eliminate that stress at its source.

1. _____
   _____

2. _____
   _____

3. _____
   _____

4. _____
   _____

5. _____
   _____

EXERCISE 1.1-J

Set behavioral goals for your first Thirty Day Block. From the above list of new and improved behaviors, commit to four that you will focus on in the upcoming month. Try to pick at least one from each category F, G, H, and I. Record your new and improved behaviors in the Thirty Day Block template shown on page 93.

EXERCISE 1.2
YOUR FIRST THIRTY DAY BLOCK

Since you are beginning your first thirty day block, it is important for you to identify your behavioral goals for the upcoming month, as noted at the end of the last section. If you have not already done so, please refer to the template on page 93, and write down your goals for your first 30 days. You might consider photocopying a blank template and filing it away for future use in case you run out of worksheets in this book.

At any time you finish a thirty day block, complete the worksheet referable to that block. Then set goals for your next thirty day block. You do not need to make it to the end of a chapter or section in your workbook prior to completing your thirty-day assessment. The point is for you to go at your own pace.

EXERCISE 1.2-A

Learn to eat small portions of food with full satisfaction.

One warning about this exercise: I will explain in taste-bud-tantalizing detail how you should eat with enjoyment. Therefore, if you're not hungry now, skip this exercise and come back to it when you *are* hungry. Otherwise, ironically, I might tempt you to eat!

A. **Determine if you are truly physically hungry.** Differentiate your psychological or emotional cravings from the physical need to eat food. (If you need help with this, review the Apple Test and other methods for distinguishing true vs. false hunger in chapter four of the main book.)

B. **If you are truly hungry, decide what food you are hungry for.** Start to imagine how different foods will taste and feel in your mouth. Are you in the mood to crunch away on snack food? Or are you in the mood for some warm, soothing soup or hot chocolate? Do you want a sweet treat like ice cream? Or a hearty meal like chicken and dumplings? Try to determine the exact food that will satisfy you both physically and emotionally.

C. **Decide on the portion size.** Maybe you will take a "half" portion or less, compared to your previous portion size. Or maybe you will take one or two fist-size quantities of food, depending on the type of food and other factors, such as your degree of hunger, your lean body mass, your exercise level, and so on.

D. **Don't go back for seconds.** Instead of putting only a few slivers of food on your plate and then going back for another sliver every three minutes, take your entire portion of one or two fists full of food at once. Put it all on the plate so you can see it all together and get an honest assessment of how much you're eating. When you eat in a piecemeal manner, eating fourteen individual slivers of cake each time you pass through the kitchen, you underestimate your true portion size. In addition, make sure you have enough to be able to leave at least one bite of every food on your plate.

E. **Create the right eating environment.** Just as you may have a special place in your home where you like to pray, designate a special place to eat, like at the kitchen table. Or maybe even at the "special" dining room table. Avoid eating in those places where you previously ate without thinking, for example, in the car, standing over the kitchen sink, at the counter, in front of the refrigerator, or while watching television. When you sit down to eat, light candles if you want to make your meal extra special. Tune out surrounding stimuli. Turn off the television and the radio.

F. **Remember the Provider of the food and pray.** For a moment, reflect on the wonder and the beauty of the food God gave you and then pray to him, either aloud or silently. Give him thanks not only for the food itself but also for the renewed attitude that allows you to feast on it without guilt. Ask him to help you know exactly when to stop eating, as well. Your prayer will also help you to become calm and focused.

G. **Eat with pleasure.** After you pray, go ahead and start eating. As you eat, *pay attention* to your meal. Don't rush your eating to get rid of the evidence, because you don't have to hide the fact you're eating, even if the food is fattening. You have as much right to good food as anyone else. Eat slowly and savor each morsel, drinking sips of water in between bites, and thanking God for the freedom from bondage. Put your fork down in between bites. Concentrate on the taste and texture of the food in your mouth at that moment, and thank God for it as you eat.

H. **Take a break from eating.** By now, depending on the volume you ate, you might choose to stop eating for a while. Wrap the rest of your food and save it for the next time you feel real hunger pangs, if you even want it then. I hope you prolonged the eating experience as long as possible to optimize your satisfaction and to allow your stomach the greatest opportunity to register the food. You can always finish your meal the next time you're hungry.

I. **Stop eating when you barely begin to feel the food in your stomach.** At first, it may be difficult to judge when you feel this sensation because you may be out-of-touch with your internal signals. However, it's not the end of the world if you misjudge. If you undershoot and eat too little, it just means that you will become hungry again sooner rather than later. If you overshoot and eat too much, it will take longer before you become hungry again. Don't get bogged down in the technical details of how much to eat, or it will detract from your joy and satisfaction in eating. Get out of your head and get into your body!

J. **Thank God for the joy and satisfaction from the meal, and then move on to other thoughts.** When you are hungry again, acknowledge your hunger pangs, but allow yourself to become distracted until they grow to the point where you'd eat an apple (mild to moderate hunger). At that point, repeat the process of identifying what you want to eat and then feed your hunger again, just as God intended.

EXERCISE 1.2-B

Record your experience with Exercise 1.2-A in the space below.

_____

_____

_____

_____

_____

_____

_____

EXERCISE 1.2-C

Guided Relaxation Exercise. Listen to one of the CD recordings, "Godly Affirmations for Weight Loss." You will need to find a quiet place and ensure to the best of your ability that you will not be interrupted. Afterward, record your insights here.

_____

_____

_____

_____

_____

_____

_____

EXERCISE 1.2-D

Find or start an Eden Diet support group.
It would be very helpful for you to join with like-minded believers as you proceed through the Eden Diet. That way you can support and encourage each other in your Christian walk, as the Bible recommends.

For help in finding or joining an Eden Diet support group in your area, visit www.TheEdenDiet.com.

EXERCISE 1.2-E

Eden Diet group prayer requests.
One way to succeed on the Eden Diet is to get your mind off your weight issues and onto more positive and constructive thoughts. Do that by focusing on how you can help other people. Pray for them. Serve them.

At your next Eden Diet group meeting, record the other members' prayer requests, and then pray for them in between meetings. These requests need not be limited to matters of weight control. You will find space to record prayer requests at the end of this workbook on page 146.

EXERCISE 1.2-F

End-of-chapter notes. Any time you receive additional insights beyond the questions that I ask, make an entry into the journal pages found at the end of each chapter. The information may come from the information I present, by God's revelation through your prayer, from what others say at your meetings, or from observations that pop into your head as you go about your daily business.

Carry your workbook or a separate journal with you at all times. That way, when you receive a revelation, you can write it down immediately so you don't forget it. If it does not fit into a particular chapter, record it in the journal pages provided it the end of this book or in a separate journal.

NOTES:

_____

_____

_____

_____

_____

_____

_____

_____

_____

_____

_____

_____

_____

_____

_____

_____

_____

_____

_____

_____

_____

_____

_____

_____

_____

_____

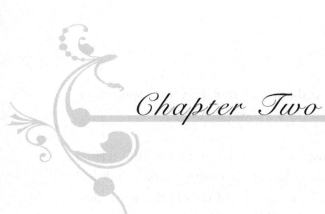

Chapter Two

Say *Good-bye* to the Diet Mentality

Begin the exercises in this chapter with the following prayer:

"Heavenly Father, clear my mind of all the myths I have come to believe about losing weight. Take my mind off of nutrition and dieting dogma and direct me to the truth. I'm tired of being misled by worldly wisdom. I want Your wisdom now. Free me from dieting bondage. Also, please speak to my heart and purify my motives for being on this plan. I want to love and respect myself as I am, and I want to lose weight to glorify You. Thank You for Your mercy and love. Amen."

In the space below, record your insights and questions from your reading of chapter 2 in *The Eden Diet*:

_____

_____

_____

_____

_____

_____

_____

WORDS OF WISDOM

▶ "To promise not to do a thing is the surest way in the world to make a body want to go and do that very thing." — Mark Twain, *The Adventures of Tom Sawyer*, 1876

▶ "Reality check: you can never, ever, use weight loss to solve problems that are not related to your weight. At your goal weight or not, you still have to live with yourself and deal with your problems. You will still have the same husband, the same job, the same kids, and the same life. Losing weight is not a cure for life." — Phillip C. McGraw, *The Ultimate Weight Solution: The 7 Keys to Weight Loss Freedom*, 2003

EXERCISE 2.1
WHAT DO YOU EXPECT FROM WEIGHT LOSS?

When I ask patients why they want to go on diets, they usually say things like, "I want to look and feel better," or "I think it will ease my joint pain." While those reasons are valid and rational, I believe some people have deeper, unconscious reasons for wanting to lose weight. Unfortunately, many of those reasons are wildly unrealistic and set dieters up for dissatisfaction and failure, no matter how much weight they lose.

If you want to feel satisfied by this program, you will need to have realistic expectations about what it can do for you.

EXERCISE 2.1-A

Take time to think about what false expectations you might have from weight loss. Read the following questions, and then pray about them before you record your responses.

- In the past, I dieted so I could be more _____ , feel more _____ , and have more _____ .

- I diet so I can feel that I am in control of _____ _____ .

- In the past, when I was on a diet that was going well, I felt that I was more
  1. _____
  2. _____ , and
  3. _____ .

- If I could lose weight, [name a specific person or people] _____ _____ would think I am more 1. _____ _____ , and
  2. _____ .

❧ If I could lose weight, [name a specific person or people]

_____ would finally do the

_____ following things for me:

_____

_____ .

❧ In the past, when I was thinner, I believed people _____ me more.

❧ In the past, when I was thinner, I believed people _____ me less.

❧ In the past, when I was thinner, I _____ myself more.

❧ In the past, when I was thinner, I _____ myself less.

❧ In the past, as long as I focused on dieting, I avoided thinking about _____ ,
which is what really bothered me deep down.

❧ In the future, when I become thinner, I expect to feel _____ .

❧ In the future, when I become thinner, I expect to have _____ .

❧ In the future, when I become thinner, I will be able to _____ .

I hope this exercise helped you to realize if you may have infused the notion of dieting with unrealistic meaning and expectations.

If you think losing weight will fix all your problems, you're in for a rude awakening. No matter how much weight you lose, you will still have problems, and you will still be tempted to feel dissatisfied with your life and those around you. That's just part of having fallen from grace back in Eden. In reality, satisfaction and happiness are states of mind, not states of the body.

Dieting may boost your self-confidence and self-esteem in the short run, but it does not solve the underlying emotional and spiritual problems that led you to gain weight to begin with. It doesn't solve your relationship problems, it doesn't give you greater power and control in life, and it doesn't make people love or respect you more. Only God can help you with all that.

Exercise 2.1-B

In the space below, record your insights about your unconscious expectations from this or any reducing diet. Explain how your unconscious expectations may have been unrealistic.

_____

_____

_____

_____

_____

Exercise 2.1-C

In the space below, write a letter to God—a prayer. Ask Him to help you have the right motives for losing weight—God-centered rather than self-centered reasons. For example, ask to glorify Him, to be a living testimony to His mercy, to become healthier so you can do more for Him, to lose weight because your body is His temple, etc. Be specific. Incorporate those thoughts into your everyday prayers as well.

_____

_____

_____

_____

_____

_____

_____

_____

_____

Exercise 2.1-D

Pray and meditate on what is *reasonable* to expect from this reducing plan. In the space below, record those more reasonable expectations.

_____

_____

_____

_____

_____

_____

_____

_____

_____

_____

EXERCISE 2.1-E

Action point. This week, pray that God opens your mind to the truth regarding why you have struggled with weight control issues. Ask if you have looked to dieting to be your crutch when God should have been your crutch. Also recognize His endless mercy and love, and that He will help you to overcome those obstacles if only you seek His help. Record God's response to you here:

_____

_____

_____

_____

_____

_____

_____

_____

_____

_____

Action point. Review the behavioral goals you set in this month's Thirty Day Block. Have you adopted healthier behaviors? Assess your progress according to the checklist below:

- ☐ Do you wait for true hunger pangs before you eat?

- ☐ Do you let your hunger build, or do you eat at the first, tiny little sensation that you feel under your breast bone?

- ☐ Do you eat much smaller portions than you once thought was "normal"?

- ☐ Do you leave food on your plate?

- ☐ Do you perform strengthening exercises (with light weights)?

- ☐ Do you stretch?

- ☐ Do you perform aerobic exercise to increase your heart rate?

If you are not doing those things consistently, re-commit. Start right now. Wait until you're hungry before you eat. Eat smaller portions. Exercise for at least twenty minutes three times a week. Increase your exercise intensity and/or duration as tolerated. Remember, faith without action is dead. Show through your *actions* that you love God and the temple He created.

WORDS OF WISDOM

▶ "Probably nothing in the world arouses more false hopes than the first four hours of a diet." —Dan Bennett

EXERCISE **2.2**
GENDER ROLES AND BODY WEIGHT

EXERCISE **2.2-A**

Women and body weight

Sometimes we unconsciously use our excess weight to speak for us. For example, in the workplace, if a woman wants to feel that she is taken seriously, she might use her excess weight to desexualize herself. Through it, she broadcasts that she is "one of the guys" rather than a "piece of meat." It might even make her feel larger and more powerful than her male colleagues.

On the other hand, excess weight can make a woman feel less threatened sexually. Since people often look right past fat women to ogle the thin, sexy ones, her weight would make her "invisible," in a sense. She wouldn't be the object of the disgusting thoughts of all the perverts out there.

In some cases, a woman's weight might be her means of rebellion. Perhaps certain people, maybe her parents or her spouse, put undue pressure on her to be slim. Maybe fatness is her way to say, "Don't tell me what to do."

There is no right or wrong answer regarding what your weight might mean to you. It's all about your perceptions. If you think your excess body weight is providing something you need, then you might miss it when it's gone.

In general, you would be well served to try to identify what perks you derived from your excess body weight, because once you lose weight, you might need a replacement crutch. In case your large size screams, "Stay away," or "I'm not going to do what you say," then find a way to say that in a more healthy way, or ask God to help change the way you feel.

EXERCISE **2.2-B**

Men and body weight

Whereas some women express that they are afraid of receiving unwanted sexual attention if they lose weight, most men are confused by this notion and say, "What sexual attention is unwanted?" I have to *explain* to them that we women feel more vulnerable because we know we can be physically overtaken by a man who finds us attractive.

Regarding issues of sexuality, the men I surveyed uniformly said they would be more likely to feel empowered in a trimmer and stronger body. Or they say it doesn't matter to them at all. I don't know why I was surprised when I learned that.

It seems that men, in general, have less complex reasons for gaining weight than women do. Most of the men I counsel on weight control gain weight by eating portions that are too large and because of not exercising enough. That's it. That's their whole reason. They don't usually eat for emotional reasons as women do. At least, they don't recognize it if they do.

Even though men are reluctant to admit it, I believe some of them might derive a hidden psychological benefit from their excess weight. As is the case with some women, some men might like having a larger physical presence. It might make them feel bigger in a psychological sense—more powerful and strong.

On the other hand, their excess weight might give them an excuse for failure. "I didn't get the promotion because I am heavy." Or, "If only I were thinner, I would get more dates." Maybe being fat gives them a handy "out" if they suffer from performance anxiety.

What is performance anxiety? Men are plagued with worries that women often do not appreciate or understand, and men are not quick to divulge these worries, either. Some of the issues relevant to men include needing to feel like the protector and hero, needing to feel like an adequate provider, and needing to feel strong and powerful.

If a man has trouble living up to these perceptions of what he should be like, or if he believes he has failed, he might rely on food as a sort of crutch. Maybe he will narcotize his feelings of inadequacy by overeating, so that he is taken out of the competition altogether.

What is the cure for this erroneous thinking? The truth of God is a good place to start. If you want to understand what God wants men to be like, think about Noah. When God was fed up with us sinners and wiped out the rest of mankind in a big flood, he spared only Noah and his family so that Noah would be the prototype for future generations.

He said, "This is the account of Noah. Noah was a righteous man, blameless among the people of his time, and he walked with God" (Genesis 6:9). Apparently, God liked that Noah checked in with Him regularly, loved Him, and loved the others around him.

God did *not* say, "Noah was a tall, muscular, strong, and confident man, with a net worth of $500,000, a brand-new Lexus, lots of hair, lots of children, lots of people working for him, and a trophy wife. So I spared him."

Once you understand God's truth, you might even begin to see that your expectations of yourself may be self-imposed misperceptions of the truth, rather than what others really expect from you. In reality, you might find that your wife would be happier with your time and loving attention rather than fancy cars. At least, I hope that's what she thinks.

EXERCISE 2.2-C

In the space below, record your insights about the ways in which your excess weight might relate to your gender identity. Has your weight allowed you to broadcast any messages that served you well in the past or perhaps given you an excuse for failure in some important area of your life?

_____

_____

_____

_____

EXERCISE 2.2-D

Come up with alternative ways to broadcast that same message or fill the same need without using your body size to speak for you.

_____

_____

_____

_____

_____

_____

_____

EXERCISE 2.3
LOOK AT YOUR ATTITUDE

EXERCISE 2.3-A

On the next page you will find two blocks. In the block at the top of the page, make a list of all your attitudes about food, eating, dieting, fatness, and thinness. Don't judge your attitudes; just write them down as you think of them.

You might write things like: "I hate my fat." "I just don't have the willpower." "My fat is what drove my boyfriend away." "I'm too weak to stay on diets." "I have a sweet tooth."

On the other hand, maybe you have positive beliefs, like: "I am ready to turn this problem over to God." "My body is His temple." "I want to set a better example for my children." Whatever your attitudes are, write them down, both the positive and the negative if you have mixed feelings, and try to be honest. Write as many as you can.

In block on the bottom of the page, write down what you think *God* would say in response to your attitudes. Make each number correspond to the number in the block above. For example, if you wrote "I hate my fat," on line one in the top block, then you might write as God's response, "God loves my fat because it's part of me" on line one in the bottom block.

When you try to discern what God's reply might be, remember His nature: He is merciful and loving and cares about you deeply. He is not concerned with trivial things like body weight, but He is concerned about you being in bondage to it.

When you have filled in all the blanks, take a big, bold marker, cross out the negative remarks you wrote, and write the word LIES right over those statements. In other words, capture your critical, merciless, negative, incorrect, fattening, ungodly thoughts, and then literally reject them in favor of the truth—God's mercy, love, and grace.

Then, circle the entire bottom block and write "TRUTH." But in this case, write the word "truth" in the margin. After all, you want to be able to read God's truth over and over again without hindrances.

Your Attitudes About Body Weight, Food, and Dieting:

1. _____
2. _____
3. _____
4. _____
5. _____
6. _____
7. _____
8. _____
9. _____
10. _____

How God Would Correct Your Attitudes (Remember that He is all about love and mercy and grace):

1. _____
2. _____
3. _____
4. _____
5. _____
6. _____
7. _____
8. _____
9. _____
10. _____

EXERCISE 2.3-B

Meditate on and pray about the last exercise. Did you uncover any areas where your perceptions may differ from God's truth? If so, what were they?

_____

_____

_____
_____
_____

EXERCISE 2.3-C

What will be your main obstacle(s) to giving up traditional dieting?

_____
_____
_____
_____

EXERCISE 2.3-D

How do you plan to overcome your obstacle(s)?

_____
_____
_____
_____

EXERCISE 2.3-E

Memorize the following Scripture verse:
▶ "So whether you eat or drink or whatever you do, do it all for the glory of God" (1 Corinthians 10:31). (In other words, dedicate your weight loss to Him too.)

EXERCISE 2.4
YOU WANT WHAT YOU THINK YOU CAN'T HAVE EVEN MORE

We all know that eating properly results in weight loss. The problem is even though we want to be perfect, we are not. Most of us are unable to eat like saints indefinitely. We put a lot of pressure on ourselves to do what's right because it's right, but our sinful nature eventually makes us fall off the wagon and overeat.

Ironically, when we diet, we plant the seeds of our own failure at weight control. We cut out all the fattening, delicious food that brings us pleasure and makes us happy, and we eat only the healthy, low-calorie food that we feel we "should" eat.

On the surface, it sounds reasonable. But the result is that we covet the fattening food that we tried to abstain from to begin with, and then we over-eat it.

If you have gone on traditional diets for any length of time, I am quite sure you know what I am talking about.

EXERCISE 2.4-A

Explain the psychological benefits of eating treats occasionally (in small amounts and only when hungry) while on a reducing diet. For example, how might it help you reestablish that you are the boss over the food?

_____

_____

_____

_____

_____

❧ How might it help ease your impulses to binge?

_____

_____

_____

❧ How might it cause you to feel more satisfied by the food you eat?

_____

_____

_____

EXERCISE 2.4-B

Memorize the following Scripture verses. Write them on note cards and take them with you. When you have a free moment, look at them and meditate on them.

▶ "Therefore I tell you, do not worry about your life, what you will eat or drink; or about your body, what you will wear. Is not life more important than food, and the body more important than clothes?" (Matthew 6:25).

▶ "For the kingdom of God is not a matter of eating and drinking, but of righteousness, peace and joy in the Holy Spirit" (Romans 14:17).

EXERCISE 2.5
HOW DIETING AFFECTS YOUR EMOTIONS

EXERCISE 2.5-A

Summarize how you believe dieting and *successfully* losing weight might affect your emotions and self-esteem.

_____

_____

_____

_____

_____

EXERCISE 2.5-B

Summarize how *failure* at dieting negatively affects your emotions (e.g. depression, anxiety about food, etc.) and how it affects your self-esteem.

_____

_____

_____

_____

_____

EXERCISE 2.5-C

Do you want your emotions and self-esteem to *continue* being tied to your body weight and eating habits? Of course, you don't. Then, write a letter to God, asking Him to help you dissociate your self-worth from your success or failure at controlling your weight. Ask Him to help you *feel* worthy because you are His child. You don't just need to *know* the truth; you need to *feel* the truth.

_____

_____

_____

_____

_____

_____

_____

_____

_____

_____

_____

_____

_____

EXERCISE 2.6
BODY IMAGE

Do you know what your body looks like? How often do you just stare into the mirror at your face and almost ignore the fact that there is anything below your neck? Do you buy tent-like clothes to hide your figure because you're embarrassed about it? Do you truly know how big or small you are? When is the last time you actually looked at your body in a mirror?

It's sad that we are driven to feel ashamed of our bodies. And it's sad that the world encourages it. Constantly, we are exposed to impossible-to-achieve, air-brushed, silicone-enhanced, computer-enhanced images of perfect-looking people in advertising. It's all around us on billboards, on television, on magazine covers. It even goes right down to the shapes of our dolls and action figures.

Now is the time to change that. We must stop idolizing those images. We must take the advertising messages captive, sweep them away, and replace them with the truth.

We must strive to see ourselves as God sees us. The truth is God made us in His image in the beginning, and even though we strayed from our physical ideal, He still loves us just as we are, right down to our every last lump and bump of cellulite.

But God also loves us too much to leave us overweight and in bondage to food. Being overweight makes us unhappy and sick, and it prevents us from carrying out the work that He laid out for us in the beginning.

EXERCISE 2.6-A

If you want to feel happier, learn to appreciate what you already have. In the space below, list ten things that you love about your body, and then thank God for them.

1. _____

2. _____

3. _____

4. _____

5. _____

6. _____

7. _____

8. _____

9. _____

10. _____

EXERCISE 2.6-B

Learn to appreciate the differences between our body shapes. If God wanted us to all have the same body weight, He probably would have made us all the same color and height too. In the space below, write a prayer that asks God to help you accept yourself and each other at any weight, large or small.

_____

_____

_____

_____

EXERCISE 2.6-C

Mirror work. Remove your clothing to your level of comfort and study your appearance in the mirror. Focus on your body in the areas below your neck. Study each little lump and bump, front and back. Try to see your body through God's eyes—with love and acceptance. As you look at your body, say aloud, "Lord, thank You for loving my body just as it is, unconditionally—every inch of it. It is Your temple. Help me think of it the same as You do, and help me treat it the way you want me to. Thank You, Lord."

EXERCISE 2.6-D

Memorize the following Scripture verse.

"Woe to him who quarrels with his Maker, to him who is but a potsherd among the potsherds on the ground. Does the clay say to the potter, 'What are you making?' Does your work say, 'He has no hands'?" (Isaiah 45:9).

EXERCISE 2.7
ESCAPE FROM BONDAGE TO FOOD

EXERCISE 2.7-A

Answer the following questions to determine if you're in bondage to food.

🍀 What thought is most likely to get you to jump out of bed in the morning? (e.g., "Pancakes!" or "Oh no! I'm late for work!" or "This is the day the Lord has made . . .")

_____

_____

🍀 Do you think about food when you're not hungry?

_____

🍀 Do you feel out of control around certain foods, so that you can't eat just a little of them without overdoing it? If so, what are those foods?

_____

_____

🍀 Approximately how many minutes do you spend each day thinking about and lamenting over what you ate, how much you weigh, how much you gained or lost, or what you might eat at the next meal?

_____

🍀 Approximately how many minutes do you spend each day reading cookbooks, talking about new recipes, looking for new recipes, or watching cooking shows?

_____

🍀 For comparison, how much time you spend each day reading Scripture, meditating on God, serving Him, worshipping Him, and praying?

_____

🍀 Have body weight issues caused you to think about yourself more than others? If so, how might that keep you from representing or serving God to the best of your ability?

_____

🍀 Do you worry about what you will or will not eat at social events?

_____

🍀 Do you try to control your eating by planning what and how much you will eat at upcoming meals?

_____

🍀 Do you feel that you have an addiction to food?

_____

❧ Do you have an "all or nothing" attitude about eating certain foods?

_____

❧ Do you ever binge after a period of restraint?

_____

❧ On an unconscious level, you may believe and act like food has control over you. But what do you think God would tell you about that? What is the real pecking order—who is Lord over you and what are you lord over?

_____

_____

EXERCISE 2.7-B

What did you learn from thinking about the above questions?

_____

_____

_____

_____

_____

_____

_____

_____

_____

_____

EXERCISE 2.7-C

Memorize the following Scripture verses.

▶ "Jesus answered, 'It is written: "Man does not live on bread alone, but on every word that comes from the mouth of God"'" (Matthew 4:4).

▶ "Jesus answered, 'It is written: "Worship the Lord your God and serve him only"'" (Luke 4:8).

❧ ""No one can serve two masters. Either he will hate the one and love the other, or he will be devoted to the one and despise the other" (Matthew 6:24).

EXERCISE 2.7-D

Pray for help to escape from bondage to food

> *"Heavenly Father, please reveal if I have offered myself in bondage to food. Are there certain foods that I feel I am afraid of eating because I feel a lack of control over them? Do I have an 'all or nothing' attitude about eating them? Do I obsess about food and then binge? If that flawed thinking is part of my problem, then please help me to think and act right. Please engrain the truth in me, that You are Lord over me and with Your help I can once again be the boss over the food. Teach me how to eat any food, even food I was once afraid of, in a way that would be acceptable—even pleasing—to You. Thank You, Lord. Amen."*

EXERCISE 2.7-E

Action point. What actions can you take this week to establish that you are the boss over the food and Jesus is Lord over you?

_____

_____

_____

_____

_____

_____

_____

_____

Action point. In what way could you step up your exercise program this week?

_____

_____

_____

_____

_____

EXERCISE 2.8
YOUR EXPERIENCE THUS FAR

EXERCISE 2.8-A

In the space below, record your successes and failures during your time on the Eden Diet. If you feel comfortable doing it, share them with your group or with a fellow Eden Dieter.

_____

_____

_____

_____

_____

_____

_____

_____

_____

EXERCISE 2.8-B

Questions and concerns. In the space below, record your questions, concerns, difficulties, and frustrations during your time on the Eden Diet. If you feel comfortable, share those with your group or with a fellow Eden Dieter.

_____

_____

_____

_____

EXERCISE 2.8-C

Guided Relaxation Exercise. Listen to one of the "Godly Affirmations for Weight Loss" recordings. Afterward, record your insights here.

_____

_____

_____

EXERCISE2.8-D

End-of-chapter journal

Chapter Three

There Is No *Bad* Food

Begin the exercise in this chapter with the following prayer:

"Dear Lord, show me what it means to eat to Your glory, as Paul alluded to in 1 Corinthians 10:31. Help me to receive food as a special gift from You and to eat it in a way that is pleasing to You. Free me from guilt when I indulge in rich, delicious food, and increase my satisfaction so that I don't even want to overeat. Help me to view my self-discipline as being an offering to You, and help me to become less focused on food and more focused on You. Amen."

In the space below, record your insights and questions from your reading of chapter 3 in *The Eden Diet*:

_____

_____

_____

_____

_____

_____

_____

_____

CHAPTER SUMMARY

In the New Covenant, God gave us all foods to enjoy in moderation. That's why Jesus said in Matthew 6:25 that we shouldn't worry about what we eat. He also said (in reference to food offered to idols), "What goes into a man's mouth does not make him 'unclean,' but what comes out of his mouth, that is what makes him 'unclean'" (Matthew 15:11). What we eat is just not that important to God.

Yet we spend so much time worrying about what we should or shouldn't eat. We spend so much time on it, in fact, that it can become a bad thing—an obsession—a distraction from Him.

My aim in this section is to help you relax your control over the type of food you eat so you can accept any food as a gift from God. I'd like to help you eat even the fattening foods you are afraid of overeating. That way, you can better escape bondage from them and refocus on Him.

However, in all fairness, it would not be a good idea for you to overdo it on the junk food. Paul said, "Everything is permissible for me"—but not everything is beneficial" (1 Corinthians 6:12). Even though you're not forbidden by the New Covenant to eat ice cream for dinner, it may not be a good idea for you to do that on a regular basis; you might get sick.

The trick will be finding the right balance, and I'll help you do that.

The exception is, if you are ill, you must ignore what I say and eat the kind of diet your doctor advises.

WORDS OF WISDOM

► "The only time to eat diet food is while you're waiting for the steak to cook."—Julia Child

► "Red meat is *not* bad for you. Now, blue-green meat, *that's* bad for you!"—Tommy Smothers

► "The biggest seller is cookbooks and the second is diet books—how not to eat what you've just learned how to cook."—Andy Rooney

EXERCISES
ASSESS YOUR ATTITUDES ABOUT DIET FOOD

EXERCISE 3-A

Check those that apply to you.

☐ I am afraid of fattening food, so I try to eat diet food as much as possible.

☐ Often, I eat when I am not hungry. Eating diet food at those times helps me to feel less guilty.

☐ No matter how good the diet food tastes, I still feel that it's inferior to the real thing, and I end up feeling dissatisfied.

☐ Sometimes, feeling dissatisfied leads me to eat extra servings of the diet food, or it leads me to eat other foods as well.

☐ I feel guilty when I eat "normal" food, especially in public.

☐ When eating at restaurants, I tend to order low-calorie food like salads and grilled chicken entrees, mostly because I think other people will judge me.

☐ When I eat diet food, I feel that I am making up for my past overeating mistakes. It makes help me to feel less guilty about being out of control when it comes to food.

☐ I'm afraid that if I eat non-diet food, I will gain even more weight.

☐ If the label says, "low-fat," "low-sugar," or "low-calorie," I let my guard down and eat extra.

☐ I often eat diet snacks right out of the box, automatically and mindlessly.

Exercise 3-B

What did you learn from exercise 3-A?

_____

_____

_____

_____

_____

Exercise 3-C

What will be your main obstacles to giving up diet food? In particular, notice if it is difficult for you to stop eating when the food is particularly delicious. If that's the case, hang on. In exercise 4-E, I will give you a handy tool to beat that urge.

_____

_____

_____

_____

_____

_____

EXERCISE 3-D

How will you overcome those obstacles?

_____

_____

_____

_____

EXERCISE 3-E

Memorize the following Scripture verse"

▶   "But food does not bring us near to God; we are no worse if we do not eat, and no better
if we do" (1 Corinthians 8:8).

EXERCISE 3-F

Action Point #1. The next time you're at the grocery store, read the list of ingredients on the low-fat
version as well as the regular version of any food you choose. Check to see if there are monoglycerides
and/or diglycerides in the product. Notice if those additives fall high on the ingredients list. If they
do, the food may not be low-fat. Record your insights from this exercise in the space below.

_____

_____

_____

_____

_____

Action Point #2. At the grocery store, examine products that are called low-sugar or no-added-sugar
and compare them to similar products that do not make those claims. Compare the number of calories and grams of total sugars. Notice if the calorie count is only marginally lower for the low-sugar
or low-fat product. Record your findings below.

_____

_____

_____

_____

Action Point #3. Try to keep a running estimate of how much money you're saving by eating normal food instead of diet food. Consider bringing that money to the altar as an offering to God or putting it to some other good use. Maybe send it to a hunger relief fund. How much money do you think you saved this week by eating small portions of normal food instead of diet food?

_____

_____

_____

_____

EXERCISE 3-G

In the space below, record your successes and failures as you have tried to put chapter 3 of _The Eden Diet_ into practice. If you feel comfortable doing it, share them with your group or with a fellow Eden Dieter.

_____

_____

_____

_____

EXERCISE 3-H

Questions and Concerns. In the space below, record your questions, concerns, difficulties, and frustrations as you tried to put chapter 3 into practice. If you feel comfortable, share them with your group or with a fellow Eden Dieter.

_____

_____

_____

_____

EXERCISE 3-I

Guided Relaxation Exercise. Listen to one of the "Godly Affirmations for Weight Loss" recordings. Afterward, record your insights here.

_____

_____

_____

EXERCISE 3-J
End-of-Chapter Notes

_____

_____

_____

_____

_____

_____

_____

_____

_____

_____

_____

_____

_____

_____

_____

_____

_____

_____

_____

_____

_____

PART Two

The **EDEN DIET**
(how to eat *normal* food and get skinny)

Chapter Four

Rediscover Your
Hunger Signals

Begin the exercise in this chapter with the following prayer:

"Heavenly Father, I trust You. I believe You planted a tremendous capacity for healing into my body, and I need Your help to find it. Help me attune to my hunger and fullness signals so I can lose weight and be a living testimony to Your healing grace. Amen."

In the space below, record your insights and questions from your reading of chapter 4 in *The Eden Diet*:

_____

_____

_____

_____

_____

_____

_____

_____

_____

WORDS OF WISDOM

▶ "A good meal ought to begin with hunger." — French Proverb

CHAPTER SUMMARY

Your bodily sensations are your compass when it comes to eating. If you feel the impulse to eat, wait a while and try to discern if you actually feel hunger pangs. If not, you are probably experiencing false hunger (emotional, mental, or spiritual). In that case, eating will not solve your problem. It will only create different problems. Obey your God-given bodily signals instead of your impulses.

Exercises
HOW TO READ YOUR HUNGER PANGS

EXERCISE 4-A

Start by attuning to your body's messages in general. Lie down and relax, and try to pay attention to how you feel physically. Are you tired? Nervous? Thirsty? Hungry? Achy? Relaxed? Fully feel those sensations without letting your mind wander. In the space below, record what your body is trying to tell you it needs, if anything.

_____

_____

_____

_____

_____

_____

_____

EXERCISE 4-B

Let yourself become hungry by abstaining from eating for a period of many hours. In the interim while you wait, get busy and become preoccupied with other activities. Probably, after many hours pass, you will begin to feel hungry. If you have difficulty identifying whether or not you're hungry, review the material in chapter 4 of *The Eden Diet*.

Once hunger pangs set in, notice how they come and go over time. Tune into the *emotions* you feel when you're hungry. Sit with those emotions for a while and notice what happens or what doesn't happen. Find ways to become distracted, and notice if your feelings about hunger change. Record your revelations about the emotions you connect with hunger in the space below:

_____

_____

_____

_____

_____

_____

EXERCISE 4-C

Action Point. If you are not losing weight, reduce your portion sizes even further. That will allow you to become hungry more frequently, which will give you more practice at tuning in to your body's messages regarding how you're supposed to eat. Notice how mastering this sensation impacts your feelings about eating. Write down how your attitudes and feelings about hunger have changed since you confronted it head-on.

_____

_____

_____

_____

_____

_____

EXERCISE 4-D

What do you think will be your main obstacles to attuning to your hunger pangs and eating smaller portions of food?

_____

_____

_____

_____

_____

_____

EXERCISE 4-E

Action Point. When you feel the urge to eat large portions of food, capture that thought and hold it hostage. Then, close your eyes and picture the urge as being an actual person—a *child*. See the urge as an immature, little toddler that is throwing a temper tantrum. The toddler wants to eat food that you, as the wise, mature adult, know is bad for it. In your mind, talk to the child and tell it what a perfect, loving parent would say. Say that eating extra food just because it tastes good leads to sickness and disease. And, promise that the child can have a little bit of that food later, when his or her body actually needs food—when he or she is *hungry*. Now, in your own words, write down what you will tell that child the very next time he or she throws a tantrum over food.

_____

_____

_____

_____

_____

_____

_____

_____

_____

_____

_____

_____

_____

_____

_____

_____

_____

_____

EXERCISE 4-F

In the space below, record your successes and failures as you have tried to put chapter 4 of *The Eden Diet* into practice. If you feel comfortable doing it, share them with your group or with a fellow Eden Dieter.

_____

_____

_____

_____

_____

_____

_____

EXERCISE 4-G

Memorize the following Scripture verse:

▶ "Blessed are those who hunger and thirst for righteousness, for they will be filled" (Matthew 5:6).

EXERCISE 4-H

Questions and Concerns. In the space below, record your questions, concerns, difficulties, and frustrations as you tried to put chapter 4 into practice. If you feel comfortable, share them with your group or with a fellow Eden Dieter.

_____

_____

_____

_____

EXERCISE 4-I

Guided Relaxation Exercise. Listen to one of the "Godly Affirmations for Weight Loss" recordings. Afterward, record your insights here.

_____

_____

_____

_____

EXERCISE 4-J

End-of-Chapter Notes

Chapter Five

Feel *More* Satisfied by *Less* Food

Begin the exercises in this chapter with the following prayer:

"Dear Lord, help me understand what it means to eat to Your glory, as Paul said in 1 Corinthians 10:31. That way, I can be more satisfied by less food. Help me slow down when I eat. Let me savor the food and appreciate it as being a precious gift from You. Remove the distractions and guilt that rob me of my joy. Give me the discipline to stop when my hunger pangs barely go away, and then give me a sense of overflowing fullness and satisfaction in You. Thank You, Lord. Amen."

In the space below, record your insights and questions from your reading of chapter 5 in *The Eden Diet*:

_____

_____

_____

_____

_____

_____

_____

_____

_____

CHAPTER SUMMARY

When you eat with the right attitude, you can derive more pleasure from eating less food. Eating a half or third portion without guilt brings you more joy than eating a triple portion secretly with guilt and shame.

Because you're a mature adult, you understand that sometimes the best gifts come in small packages. You should savor and enjoy your food the same way you savor and enjoy the other kinds of precious gifts that you receive in life.

Pretend your tiny cream puff is like a diamond necklace. It's small, but it's special. It's something to relish.

The exercises in this chapter will help you to develop a whole new concept of how much food is enough. The key point to remember is that you are not actually depriving yourself when you eat smaller portions. You're just delaying gratification. If you eat a third or a half of a normal portion now, you can always eat more of that same food the very next time you get hungry.

WORDS OF WISDOM

▶ "Never eat more than you can lift."—Miss Piggy.

EXERCISES
WHY DON'T YOU ENJOY YOUR FOOD?

EXERCISE 5-A

Write down the attitudes and/or emotions that interfere with your ability to truly enjoy your food. List as many as you can.

1. _____

2. _____

3. _____

4. _____

5. _____

6. _____

7. _____

8. _____

9. _____

10. _____

EXERCISE **5-B**

How can you change those factors so you derive more joy from the eating experience? Match the numbers below to those listed above.

1. _____

2. _____

3. _____

4. _____

5. _____

6. _____

7. _____

8. _____

9. _____

10. _____

EXERCISE **5-C**

Memorize the following Scripture verses:

▶ "My flesh and my heart may fail, but God is the strength of my heart and my portion forever" (Psalm 73:26).

▶ "If you find honey, eat just enough— too much of it, and you will vomit" (Proverbs 25:16).

EXERCISE **5-D**

In the space below, record your successes and failures as you have tried to put chapter 5 of *The Eden Diet* into practice. If you feel comfortable doing it, share them with your group or with a fellow Eden Dieter.

_____

_____

_____

_____

_____

_____

_____

_____

_____

_____

EXERCISE 5-E

Questions and Concerns. In the space below, record your questions, concerns, difficulties, and frustrations as you tried to put chapter 5 into practice. If you feel comfortable, share them with your group or with a fellow Eden Dieter and together brainstorm solutions.

_____

_____

_____

_____

_____

_____

_____

EXERCISE 5-F

Action point. Evaluate your attitudes about exercise. Do they match your attitudes about eating? Are you learning to exercise to the glory of God, just as you are learning to eat to the glory of God? If not, pray that God transforms your mind about exercise so that you enjoy it more. And then, act like you're already transformed and increase your exercise duration, frequency, and intensity.

_____

_____

_____

_____

_____

_____

EXERCISE 5-G

Guided Relaxation Exercise. Listen to one of the "Godly Affirmations for Weight Loss" CDs. Afterward, record your insights here.

_____

_____

_____

_____

_____

_____

EXERCISE 5-H

End-of-Chapter Notes

_____

_____

_____

_____

_____

_____

_____

_____

_____

_____

_____

_____

_____

_____

_____

_____

_____

_____

Chapter Six

The EDEN DIET in Action

Begin the exercises in this chapter with the following prayer:

"Dear Lord, please give me the strength, discipline, and desire to eat properly as an offering to You. Help me to give up the notion of willpower and rest on Your power. Make this plan second-nature to me, so that it becomes automatic and easy. Thank You for Your forgiveness and mercy. Amen."

In the space below, record your insights and questions from your reading of chapter 6 in *The Eden Diet***:**

_____

_____

_____

_____

_____

_____

_____

_____

_____

_____

CHAPTER SUMMARY

Show God you love Him through your actions. Use self-discipline and the strategies I offer for those especially challenging situations, like eating at potlucks and buffets. Be aware that some people may try to sabotage your weight loss, but be kind to them because they are probably hurting in some way too.

EXERCISES
HOW TO EAT IN CHALLENGING SITUATIONS

EXERCISE 6-A

Face your enemy. Ideally, you should minimize unnecessary temptation by not eating out too frequently. But on those occasions when you do eat at restaurants, you need strategies to help you eat properly. In the space below, list at least ten strategies for eating at restaurants. Include examples for fast food restaurants, regular ala carte restaurants, and buffets and potlucks.

1. _____
2. _____
3. _____
4. _____
5. _____
6. _____
7. _____
8. _____
9. _____
10. _____

EXERCISE 6-B

Action point. Put your strategies into practice. Eat at a restaurant. Record your experience and feelings in the space below.

_____

_____

_____

_____

_____

EXERCISE 6-C

Accumulate strategies for when you attend social situations that revolve around food.

List at least five tactful ways to say no when someone offers you food that you're not hungry for.

1. _____
2. _____
3. _____
4. _____
5. _____

"Is that all you're going to eat?" Get ready for this question. I mean that literally! Make a list of five things you can say when you're asked "Is that all you're going to eat?" Record your responses below.

1. _____
2. _____
3. _____
4. _____
5. _____

Learn how to change the subject. Make a list of five things you can say to change the subject when a person either criticizes your weight loss method or if they talk excessively about food.

1. _____
2. _____
3. _____
4. _____
5. _____

EXERCISE 6-D

Memorize the following Scripture verses:

▶ "If you fully obey the LORD your God and carefully follow all his commands I give you today, the LORD your God will set you high above all the nations on earth" (Deuteronomy 28:1).

▶ "Don't you know that when you offer yourselves to someone to obey him as slaves, you are slaves to the one whom you obey—whether you are slaves to sin, which leads to death, or to obedience, which leads to righteousness?" (Romans 6:16).

EXERCISE 6-E

In the space below, record your successes and failures as you have tried to put chapter 6 of *The Eden Diet* into practice. If you feel comfortable doing it, share them with your group or with a fellow Eden Dieter.

_____

_____

_____

_____

_____

_____

EXERCISE 6-F

What do you think will be your main obstacles as you try to eat in social situations?

_____

_____

_____

_____

_____

EXERCISE 6-G

How do you plan to overcome these obstacles?

_____

_____

_____

_____

_____

_____

EXERCISE 6-H

Questions and Concerns. In the space below, record your questions, concerns, difficulties, and frustrations as you tried to put chapter 6 into practice. If you feel comfortable, share them with your group or with a fellow Eden Dieter.

_____

_____

_____

_____

_____

EXERCISE 6-I

Guided Relaxation Exercise. Listen to one of the "Godly Affirmations for Weight Loss" CDs. Afterward, record your insights here.

_____

_____

_____

_____

_____

EXERCISE 6-J

End-of-Chapter Journal

_____

_____

_____

_____

_____

_____

_____

_____

_____

how to *beat* temptation

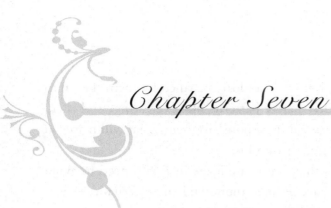

Chapter Seven

Feed Emotional Hunger the *Right* Way

Begin the exercises in this chapter with the following prayer:

"Dear Lord, please help me to recognize the emotions that trigger me to eat when I'm not actually hungry. When You believe the time is right, help me to face those emotions directly and take control over them. Teach me to engage in healthier responses to my emotions besides eating. Thank You, Lord. Amen."

In the space below, record your insights and questions from your reading of chapter 7 in *The Eden Diet*:

_____

_____

_____

_____

_____

_____

_____

_____

_____

_____

CHAPTER SUMMARY

Emotions are a normal part of the human experience, but you shouldn't be ruled by them. Learn to recognize when they are manipulating you into self-destructive patterns like overeating, and then, when possible try to experience them directly rather than eat in response to them. That will help you dissociate the learned response of eating from the emotional stimulus.

You can also compile a list of healthy distractions that you can engage in if you need to avoid feeling those emotions directly. The exception is if you have serious emotional issues. In that case, you should seek counseling to help you deal with those emotions.

WORDS OF WISDOM

▶ "If food is your best friend, it's also your worst enemy."—Edward "Grandpa" Jones, 1978

▶ "If hunger is not the problem, then eating is not the solution."—Author Unknown

EXERCISES
SEPARATING YOUR HUNGER FROM YOUR EMOTIONS

EXERCISE 7-A

When you feel the urge to eat when you're not actually hungry, try to tune in to your emotions. Do you feel bored, anxious, depressed, lonely, or tired? Try to discern the emotions that are your "triggers" for eating when you're not hungry, and then record them in your journal.

_____

_____

_____

_____

_____

EXERCISE 7-B

Make the choice to not eat when you feel your triggers. Try to feel that emotion directly instead of eating in response to it. Simply sit there and feel anxious or stressed or bored for at least ten or fifteen minutes. Embrace the emotion. Perhaps that emotion made you feel uncomfortable for a little while, but was it actually lethal? (Hint—if you are still breathing, the answer is no.) Record your experience here. What (if anything) happened when you experienced your emotions directly instead of eating in response to them?

_____

_____

_____

_____

_____

_____

_____

EXERCISE 7-C

The million dollar question: If our emotions aren't actually lethal, then why do we try to run from them rather than feel them?

_____

_____

_____

_____

_____

_____

_____

EXERCISE 7-D

There is no better comfort food than the Bread of Life. If you feel uncomfortable with your emotions, turn to God and pray when you experience them. After you pray, record your insights below.

_____

_____

_____

_____

_____

_____

_____

EXERCISE 7-E

A reasonable short-term fix is to distract yourself from your emotions when you are very uncomfortable with them. Compile a list of non-food-related, healthy activities that you can engage in when you feel uncomfortable — and then do them.

1. _____
2. _____
3. _____
4. _____
5. _____
6. _____
7. _____
8. _____
9. _____
10. _____

EXERCISE 7-F

What do you think will be your main obstacles as you try to combat emotional eating?

_____

_____

_____

_____

_____

EXERCISE 7-G

How do you plan to overcome these obstacles?

_____

_____

_____

_____

_____

EXERCISE 7-H

Memorize the following Scripture verses:

▶ "Do not let your hearts be troubled. Trust in God; trust also in me" (John 14:1).

▶ "Come to me, all you who are weary and burdened, and I will give you rest" (Matthew 11:28).

EXERCISE 7-I

In the space below, record your successes and failures as you have tried to put chapter 7 of *The Eden Diet* into practice. If you feel comfortable doing it, share them with your group or with a fellow Eden Dieter.

_____

_____

_____

_____

_____

EXERCISE 7-J

Questions and Concerns. In the space below, record your questions, concerns, difficulties, and frustrations as you tried to put chapter 7 into practice. If you feel comfortable, share them with your group or with a fellow Eden Dieter.

_____

_____

_____

_____

_____

EXERCISE 7-K

Guided Relaxation Exercise. Listen to one of the "Godly Affirmations for Weight Loss" CDs. Afterward, record your insights here.

_____

_____

_____

_____

EXERCISE 7-L

End-of-Chapter Notes

_____

_____

_____

_____

_____

_____

_____

_____

_____

_____

_____

_____

_____

_____

_____

_____

_____

_____

_____

_____

_____

_____

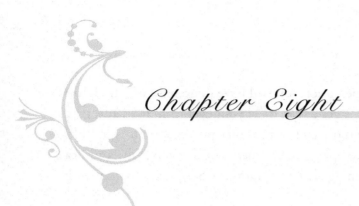

Chapter Eight

Temptation-Fighting *Tools*

Begin the exercises in this chapter with the following prayer:

"Heavenly Father, please reveal to me the places, situations, and people that trigger me to eat mindlessly or in response to my sinful desires. Help me to avoid those situations where possible, and to defeat those urges when they arise. Give me strategies that will help me defeat the enemy. Help me put the food down, mid-bite, if I am eating it without thinking. Please forgive me, help me forgive myself, and help me resist the urge to condemn myself over my past eating indiscretions. Thank You for Your infinite mercy and forgiveness. Amen."

In the space below, record your insights and questions from your reading of chapter 8 in *The Eden Diet*:

_____

_____

_____

_____

_____

_____

_____

_____

_____

CHAPTER SUMMARY

Even though you get to eat food you enjoy on the Eden Diet, you still have to exercise self-discipline. You have to guard your thoughts from inappropriate urges to eat, avert your eyes from food advertisements, close your nose when you smell food that tempts you, eat smaller portions than you'd like, deal with your emotions more directly, don't keep tempting food where you see it readily, and beat down sin by doing the opposite. Your secret weapon against temptation is Scripture. Memorize it, dwell on it, live it, and breathe it.

EXERCISES
TOOLS

EXERCISE 8-A

Name the enemy. Below I've listed common sins that typically relate to our weight loss struggles. After each one, record techniques to defeat those sinful urges. I included some blanks in case I missed a sinful desire that is relevant in your life.

1. Greed: _____

2. Pride: _____

3. Gluttony: _____

4. Sloth: _____

5. Covetousness: _____

6. Disobedience: _____

7. Idolatry: _____

8. [   ]: _____

9. [   ]: _____

10. [   ]: _____

EXERCISE 8-B

In the space below, identify the factors (emotions, situations, people, locations, events) that make you more susceptible to overeating.

1. _____

2. _____

3. _____

4. _____

5. _____

6. _____

7. _____

8. _____

9. _____

10. _____

EXERCISE 8-C

In the space below, list the corresponding ways you can counter those factors you listed above (e.g., if you eat in response to stress, list ways to eliminate your stress; if you overeat at buffet restaurants, either eat at home or choose ala carte).

1. _____

2. _____

3. _____

4. _____

5. _____

6. _____

7. _____

8. _____

9. _____

10. _____

EXERCISE 8-D

List other temptation-fighting tools that are directly relevant in your life. Hint: think about your "senses" (smell, touch, sight, taste, hearing) and how they can fool you into eating when you're not hungry. And think of how you can use avoidance. Be specific. Example: "When I go to the mall, I'll plug my nose when I walk near the food court so I won't smell the cinnamon rolls, or I'll walk the other way."

1. _____

2. _____

3. _____

4. _____

5. _____

6. _____

7. _____

8. _____

9. _____

10. _____

EXERCISE 8-E

Choose your thoughts wisely. Memorize the following Scriptures and recite them when needed to combat temptation:

▶ "Submit yourselves, then, to God. Resist the devil, and he will flee from you" (James 4:7).

▶ "Jesus answered, 'It is written: "Man does not live on bread alone, but on every word that comes from the mouth of God"'" (Matthew 4:4).

▶ "Jesus turned and said to Peter, 'Get behind me, Satan! You are a stumbling block to me; you do not have in mind the things of God, but the things of men'" (Matthew 16:23).

▶ "No temptation has seized you except what is common to man. And God is faithful; he will not let you be tempted beyond what you can bear. But when you are tempted, he will also provide a way out so that you can stand up under it" (1 Corinthians 10:13).

▶ "Blessed are you, O land whose king is of noble birth and whose princes eat at a proper time—for strength and not for drunkenness" (Ecclesiastes 10:17).

▶ "When the woman saw that the fruit of the tree was good for food and pleasing to the eye, and also desirable for gaining wisdom, she took some and ate it. She also gave some to her husband, who was with her, and he ate it" (Genesis 3:6).

▶ "There is a way that seems right to a man, but in the end it leads to death" (Proverbs 14:12).

EXERCISE 8-F

Make a list of healthy physical activities you can engage in when you're tempted to eat at the wrong time. Depending on your level of health, you may need to consult with your physician.

1. _____
2. _____
3. _____
4. _____
5. _____
6. _____
7. _____
8. _____
9. _____
10. _____

EXERCISE 8-G

Action point. Renew your commitment to exercise, gradually increasing the intensity, duration, and frequency, as recommended by your personal physician. If you are well, then work up to being able to exercise five times per week for at least 30 minutes. Include strength training (weights), aerobic exercise to increase your heart rate, and stretching exercise for flexibility. Consider obtaining professional guidance regarding what type of exercise is best for your body.

EXERCISE 8-H

In the space below, record your successes and failures as you have tried to put chapter 8 of *The Eden Diet* into practice. If you feel comfortable doing it, share them with your group or with a fellow Eden Dieter.

_____
_____
_____
_____
_____
_____

EXERCISE 8-I

Questions and Concerns. In the space below, record your questions, concerns, difficulties, and frustrations as you tried to put chapter 8 into practice. If you feel comfortable, share those with your group or with a fellow Eden Dieter.

_____

_____

_____

_____

EXERCISE 8-J

Guided Relaxation Exercise. Listen to one of the "Godly Affirmations for Weight Loss" recordings. Afterward, record your insights here.

_____

_____

_____

_____

EXERCISE 8-K

End-of-Chapter Notes

_____

_____

_____

_____

_____

_____

_____

_____

_____

_____

_____

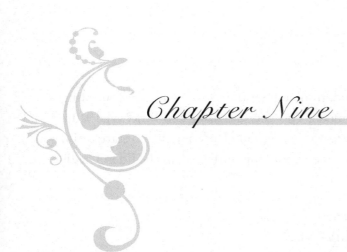

Chapter Nine

Press *On*

Begin the exercises in this chapter with the following prayer:

"Heavenly Father, please help me to forgive myself when I make mistakes, just as You forgive me. I know that perseverance is the key to success on this journey, and I need You to help me persevere. Help me to discern why I haven't lost weight if that occurs, and give me the strength to make corrections where needed. Continue to transform my mind with right thoughts about food and eating, and help me to press on toward the goal You have set for me. Thank You, Lord. Amen."

In the space below, record your insights and questions from your reading of chapter 9 in *The Eden Diet*:

_____

_____

_____

_____

_____

_____

_____

_____

_____

CHAPTER SUMMARY

If you aren't losing weight as fast as you think you should, troubleshoot the reason why. Are you eating before you become truly hungry? Are you eating too much? Are you exercising too little? Make the appropriate adjustments and keep trying. If you fall off the wagon, get right back onto it and start again. It's never too late to recover from a mistake. Keep your eyes on your long-term goal, as the Eden Diet is a life-long process. Press on.

EXERCISES
PRACTICE FORGIVENESS

EXERCISE 9-A

Do you feel differently about your eating mistakes now compared to when you were on a traditional diet? How so?

_____

_____

_____

_____

_____

_____

_____

EXERCISE 9-B

If you had difficulty losing weight at times on this plan, what adjustments did you have to make to lose weight faster?

_____

_____

_____

_____

_____

_____

_____

EXERCISE 9-C

In the space below, record your successes and failures as you have tried to put chapter 9 of *The Eden Diet* into practice. If you feel comfortable doing it, share them with your group or with a fellow Eden Dieter.

_____

_____

_____

_____

_____

_____

_____

EXERCISE 9-D

Memorize the following Scripture verses:

▶ "I can do everything through him who gives me strength" (Philippians 4:13).

▶ "Therefore, I urge you, brothers, in view of God's mercy, to offer your bodies as living sacrifices, holy and pleasing to God—this is your spiritual act of worship. Do not conform any longer to the pattern of this world, but be transformed by the renewing of your mind. Then you will be able to test and approve what God's will is—his good, pleasing and perfect will" (Romans 12:1–2).

EXERCISE 9-E

Questions and Concerns. In the space below, record your questions, concerns, difficulties, and frustrations as you tried to put chapter 9 into practice. If you feel comfortable, share them with your group or with a fellow Eden Dieter.

_____

_____

_____

_____

_____

_____

_____

EXERCISE 9-F

Action point. Write a thank You letter to God for the insight you gained through this program.

_____

_____

_____

_____

_____

_____

_____

_____

_____

_____

_____

_____

_____

EXERCISE 9-G

Guided Relaxation Exercise. Listen to one of the "Godly Affirmations for Weight Loss" recordings. Afterward, record your insights here.

_____

_____

_____

_____

_____

_____

EXERCISE 9-H

End-of-Chapter Notes

The Thirty Day Record

Block # _____   Starting Weight _____

Start Date _____   Ending Weight _____

End Date _____

STARTING MEASUREMENTS

Chest _____

Waist _____

Hips _____

Thighs _____

Arms _____

ENDING MEASUREMENTS

Chest _____

Waist _____

Hips _____

Thighs _____

Arms _____

BEHAVIORAL GOALS:

This month, I will focus on (include eating, exercise, and prayer habits as well as ways to de-stress) :

_____

_____

_____

_____

_____

END-OF-THE-MONTH REPORT: Successes and failures:

_____

_____

_____

_____

_____

_____

_____

_____

The Thirty Day Record

Block # _____   Starting Weight _____

Start Date _____   Ending Weight _____

End Date _____

STARTING MEASUREMENTS

Chest _____

Waist _____

Hips _____

Thighs _____

Arms _____

ENDING MEASUREMENTS

Chest _____

Waist _____

Hips _____

Thighs _____

Arms _____

BEHAVIORAL GOALS:

This month, I will focus on (include eating, exercise, and prayer habits as well as ways to de-stress) :

_____

_____

_____

_____

_____

END-OF-THE-MONTH REPORT: Successes and failures:

_____

_____

_____

_____

_____

_____

_____

_____

The Thirty Day Record

Block # _____   Starting Weight _____

Start Date _____   Ending Weight _____

End Date _____

STARTING MEASUREMENTS   ## ENDING MEASUREMENTS

Chest _____   Chest _____

Waist _____   Waist _____

Hips _____   Hips _____

Thighs _____   Thighs _____

Arms _____   Arms _____

BEHAVIORAL GOALS:

This month, I will focus on (include eating, exercise, and prayer habits as well as ways to de-stress) :

_____

_____

_____

_____

_____

END-OF-THE-MONTH REPORT: Successes and failures:

_____

_____

_____

_____

_____

_____

_____

_____

The Thirty Day Record

Block # _____   Starting Weight _____

Start Date _____   Ending Weight _____

End Date _____

STARTING MEASUREMENTS

Chest _____

Waist _____

Hips _____

Thighs _____

Arms _____

ENDING MEASUREMENTS

Chest _____

Waist _____

Hips _____

Thighs _____

Arms _____

BEHAVIORAL GOALS:

This month, I will focus on (include eating, exercise, and prayer habits as well as ways to de-stress) :

_____

_____

_____

_____

_____

END-OF-THE-MONTH REPORT: Successes and failures:

_____

_____

_____

_____

_____

_____

_____

_____

_____

The Thirty Day Record

Block # _____   Starting Weight _____

Start Date _____   Ending Weight _____

End Date _____

STARTING MEASUREMENTS

Chest _____

Waist _____

Hips _____

Thighs _____

Arms _____

ENDING MEASUREMENTS

Chest _____

Waist _____

Hips _____

Thighs _____

Arms _____

BEHAVIORAL GOALS:

This month, I will focus on (include eating, exercise, and prayer habits as well as ways to de-stress) :

_____

_____

_____

_____

_____

END-OF-THE-MONTH REPORT: Successes and failures:

_____

_____

_____

_____

_____

_____

_____

_____

The Thirty Day Record

Block # _____   Starting Weight _____

Start Date _____   Ending Weight _____

End Date _____

STARTING MEASUREMENTS   ## ENDING MEASUREMENTS

Chest _____   Chest _____

Waist _____   Waist _____

Hips _____   Hips _____

Thighs _____   Thighs _____

Arms _____   Arms _____

BEHAVIORAL GOALS:
This month, I will focus on (include eating, exercise, and prayer habits as well as ways to de-stress) :

_____

_____

_____

_____

_____

END-OF-THE-MONTH REPORT: Successes and failures:

_____

_____

_____

_____

_____

_____

_____

_____

The Thirty Day Record

Block # _____   Starting Weight _____

Start Date _____   Ending Weight _____

End Date _____

STARTING MEASUREMENTS

Chest _____

Waist _____

Hips _____

Thighs _____

Arms _____

ENDING MEASUREMENTS

Chest _____

Waist _____

Hips _____

Thighs _____

Arms _____

BEHAVIORAL GOALS:

This month, I will focus on (include eating, exercise, and prayer habits as well as ways to de-stress) :

_____

_____

_____

_____

_____

END-OF-THE-MONTH REPORT: Successes and failures:

_____

_____

_____

_____

_____

_____

_____

_____

The Thirty Day Record

Block # _____   Starting Weight _____

Start Date _____   Ending Weight _____

End Date _____

STARTING MEASUREMENTS   ## ENDING MEASUREMENTS

Chest _____   Chest _____

Waist _____   Waist _____

Hips _____   Hips _____

Thighs _____   Thighs _____

Arms _____   Arms _____

BEHAVIORAL GOALS:

This month, I will focus on (include eating, exercise, and prayer habits as well as ways to de-stress) :

_____

_____

_____

_____

_____

END-OF-THE-MONTH REPORT: Successes and failures:

_____

_____

_____

_____

_____

_____

_____

_____

The Thirty Day Record

Block # _____   Starting Weight _____

Start Date _____   Ending Weight _____

End Date _____

STARTING MEASUREMENTS

Chest _____

Waist _____

Hips _____

Thighs _____

Arms _____

ENDING MEASUREMENTS

Chest _____

Waist _____

Hips _____

Thighs _____

Arms _____

BEHAVIORAL GOALS:

This month, I will focus on (include eating, exercise, and prayer habits as well as ways to de-stress) :

_____

_____

_____

_____

_____

END-OF-THE-MONTH REPORT: Successes and failures:

_____

_____

_____

_____

_____

_____

_____

_____

The Thirty Day Record

Block # _____   Starting Weight _____

Start Date _____   Ending Weight _____

End Date _____

STARTING MEASUREMENTS   ## ENDING MEASUREMENTS

Chest _____   Chest _____

Waist _____   Waist _____

Hips _____   Hips _____

Thighs _____   Thighs _____

Arms _____   Arms _____

BEHAVIORAL GOALS:
This month, I will focus on (include eating, exercise, and prayer habits as well as ways to de-stress) :

_____

_____

_____

_____

_____

END-OF-THE-MONTH REPORT: Successes and failures:

_____

_____

_____

_____

_____

_____

_____

_____

The Thirty Day Record

Block # _____   Starting Weight _____

Start Date _____   Ending Weight _____

End Date _____

STARTING MEASUREMENTS   ### ENDING MEASUREMENTS

Chest _____   Chest _____

Waist _____   Waist _____

Hips _____   Hips _____

Thighs _____   Thighs _____

Arms _____   Arms _____

BEHAVIORAL GOALS:
This month, I will focus on (include eating, exercise, and prayer habits as well as ways to de-stress) :

_____

_____

_____

_____

_____

END-OF-THE-MONTH REPORT: Successes and failures:

_____

_____

_____

_____

_____

_____

_____

_____

The Thirty Day Record

Block # _____   Starting Weight _____

Start Date _____   Ending Weight _____

End Date _____

STARTING MEASUREMENTS

Chest _____

Waist _____

Hips _____

Thighs _____

Arms _____

ENDING MEASUREMENTS

Chest _____

Waist _____

Hips _____

Thighs _____

Arms _____

BEHAVIORAL GOALS:

This month, I will focus on (include eating, exercise, and prayer habits as well as ways to de-stress) :

_____

_____

_____

_____

_____

END-OF-THE-MONTH REPORT: Successes and failures:

_____

_____

_____

_____

_____

_____

_____

_____

Food Diary

AS I MENTIONED in chapter 1 of *The Eden Diet*, keeping a food diary can be counterproductive for some people. For example, if you are already losing weight on this plan, it probably means that you are beginning to eat in a more natural way, according to your bodily signals. If that is the case, you should skip over this section. It would go against the whole premise of this plan, which is to become *less* preoccupied with food.

However, if you haven't lost as much weight as you wanted to, then this exercise might help you discover the reasons why.

As you keep the diary, be sure to have the right attitude about it. Instead of thinking of it as a way to police the way you eat, as if Big Brother were watching you, think of it as a tool that God has given you so you can learn the truth. Instead of trying to be "extra good" when you keep the diary, try to let it reflect an average cross-section of your eating. You have to be honest with yourself as well as with God if you want to move forward in your Romans 12:1–2 mental makeover.

Try to record your entries immediately after you eat the food, not at the end of the day. If you delay making the entry into the diary, you may forget the emotion or situation that triggered you to eat. In addition, you may remember your meals, but you may not remember the ten or twelve little tidbits you might have eaten mindlessly during the course of the day.

In addition, record specific details about what you eat. Instead of writing, "casserole," write "one scoop of chicken enchilada casserole with corn, cheese, chilies, onions, and flour tortillas." It makes you really pay attention and embrace the little nuances of the food you're eating so that you can appreciate the food more.

As soon as you become more aware of your mindless eating habits, please stop keeping the diary. Normal eaters don't keep a food diary, and since your goal is to eat more normally, you don't have to, either. It's just an exercise to help you recognize the fattening habits you may previously have been unaware of.

Sample Food Diary

Date: _____

BREAKFAST:	WHY I ATE:	OLD HABIT OR NEW HABIT?
3/4 cup oatmeal	Hungry	New—didn't eat every bite, didn't wolf it down, paid attention.
2 t real butter		
1T brown sugar		
Water		
LUNCH:		
2½ slices pepperoni pizza	Hungry, irritable	In between. I told myself I would only have one slice, but was distracted and got more. Stressful day.
Diet lemonade		
DINNER:		
Chef salad with cheese, Turkey, veggies, croutons, Dressing	Dinnertime	Old. Wasn't hungry; ate a big lunch. Picked at salad because not hungry. Should have just waited.
Diet pop		
SNACKS:		
3 mini chocolate bars	Tired	Old. Should have rested.
Apple	Hungry	New. Enjoyed it.

Food Diary

Date: _____

BREAKFAST:	WHY I ATE:	OLD HABIT OR NEW HABIT?
LUNCH:		
DINNER:		
SNACKS:		

What I did right:

_____

_____

Where did I consume calories that I might have otherwise not counted previously? What mindless eating habits did I discover?

_____

_____

Food Diary

Date: _____

BREAKFAST:	WHY I ATE:	OLD HABIT OR NEW HABIT?
LUNCH:		
DINNER:		
SNACKS:		

What I did right:

_____

_____

Where did I consume calories that I might have otherwise not counted previously? What mindless eating habits did I discover?

_____

_____

Food Diary

Date: _____

Breakfast:	Why I ate:	Old Habit or New Habit?
Lunch:		
Dinner:		
Snacks:		

What I did right:

_____

_____

Where did I consume calories that I might have otherwise not counted previously? What mindless eating habits did I discover?

_____

_____

Food Diary

Date: _____

BREAKFAST:	WHY I ATE:	OLD HABIT OR NEW HABIT?
LUNCH:		
DINNER:		
SNACKS:		

What I did right:

_____

_____

Where did I consume calories that I might have otherwise not counted previously? What mindless eating habits did I discover?

_____

_____

Food Diary

Date: _____

Breakfast:	Why I ate:	Old Habit or New Habit?
Lunch:		
Dinner:		
Snacks:		

What I did right:

_____

_____

Where did I consume calories that I might have otherwise not counted previously? What mindless eating habits did I discover?

_____

_____

Food Diary

Date: _____

BREAKFAST:	WHY I ATE:	OLD HABIT OR NEW HABIT?
LUNCH:		
DINNER:		
SNACKS:		

What I did right:

_____

_____

Where did I consume calories that I might have otherwise not counted previously? What mindless eating habits did I discover?

_____

_____

Food Diary

Date: _____

Breakfast:	Why I ate:	Old Habit or New Habit?
Lunch:		
Dinner:		
Snacks:		

What I did right:

_____

_____

Where did I consume calories that I might have otherwise not counted previously? What mindless eating habits did I discover?

_____

_____

Food Diary

Date: _____

Breakfast:	Why I ate:	Old Habit or New Habit?
Lunch:		
Dinner:		
Snacks:		

What I did right:

_____

_____

Where did I consume calories that I might have otherwise not counted previously? What mindless eating habits did I discover?

_____

_____

Food Diary

Date: _____

BREAKFAST:	WHY I ATE:	OLD HABIT OR NEW HABIT?
LUNCH:		
DINNER:		
SNACKS:		

What I did right:

_____

_____

Where did I consume calories that I might have otherwise not counted previously? What mindless eating habits did I discover?

_____

_____

Food Diary

Date: _____

BREAKFAST:	WHY I ATE:	OLD HABIT OR NEW HABIT?
LUNCH:		
DINNER:		
SNACKS:		

What I did right:

_____

_____

Where did I consume calories that I might have otherwise not counted previously? What mindless eating habits did I discover?

_____

_____

Food Diary

Date: _____

BREAKFAST:	WHY I ATE:	OLD HABIT OR NEW HABIT?
LUNCH:		
DINNER:		
SNACKS:		

What I did right:

_____

_____

Where did I consume calories that I might have otherwise not counted previously? What mindless eating habits did I discover?

_____

_____

Food Diary

Date: _____

BREAKFAST:	WHY I ATE:	OLD HABIT OR NEW HABIT?
LUNCH:		
DINNER:		
SNACKS:		

What I did right:

_____

_____

Where did I consume calories that I might have otherwise not counted previously? What mindless eating habits did I discover?

_____

_____

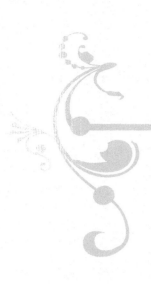

About the
Audio *Relaxation*
Exercises

I N ROMANS 12:1–2, PAUL talks about a renewing of the mind that occurs when you submit to God and let Him transform you. Applied to weight control, that means you must cooperate with God, rid your mind of the worldly notions that make you fat, and fill your mind with thoughts and ideas that are consistent with His teachings in the Bible.

You can rely on God to change your mind, but don't expect Him to do the whole thing for you. You also need to cooperate with Him and make choices that are consistent with what He is trying to do in your life.

If you do that, what happens next is amazing—your body changes in accordance with your mind-set. Once your thinking is aligned with the Word, your body automatically starts slimming down. You change from the inside out.

The reason is simple. Your thoughts about food, eating, and exercise determine your choices, and your choices determine your habits. Your habits, in turn, determine your body size.

In order to reinforce your Romans 12:1–2 renewing of the mind for weight control, I have created audio CDs that reinforce Eden Diet teachings. They are for use by you privately, whenever you feel you need to listen to them, and also for use near the end of your Eden Diet workshops. You can listen to any of the CDs at the end of any exercise in the workbook. There is no set structure to which one you should listen to at what time.

When you prepare to listen to the CDs, it's important for you to be mentally and physically ready. In a workshop setting, the group should generally break just before the meeting to allow time for members to stretch their legs, use the restroom, turn off cell phones, and adjust or change their clothing, if needed. It is also recommended that a group member place a "Please Be Quiet—Relaxation Exercise in Progress" sign on the door. And they should check the immediate area for non-group people who might cause noisy distractions and ask them to move to a different area, or at least ask them to hold their noise down.

You should allow at least twenty to thirty minutes for the exercise, so that you will be able to come out of it in the most comfortable, relaxing way.

Journal

Journal

Journal

Journal

Journal

Journal

Journal

Journal

Journal

Journal

Journal

Journal

Journal

Journal

Journal

Journal

Journal

Journal

Journal

Journal

Journal

Group Contact Information

Name:	Name:
Home Phone:	Home Phone:
Work Phone:	Work Phone:
Cell Phone:	Cell Phone:
E-mail:	E-mail:

Name:	Name:
Home Phone:	Home Phone:
Work Phone:	Work Phone:
Cell Phone:	Cell Phone:
E-mail:	E-mail:

Name:	Name:
Home Phone:	Home Phone:
Work Phone:	Work Phone:
Cell Phone:	Cell Phone:
E-mail:	E-mail:

Name:	Name:
Home Phone:	Home Phone:
Work Phone:	Work Phone:
Cell Phone:	Cell Phone:
E-mail:	E-mail:

Name:	Name:
Home Phone:	Home Phone:
Work Phone:	Work Phone:
Cell Phone:	Cell Phone:
E-mail:	E-mail:

Group Contact Information

Name:	Name:
Home Phone:	Home Phone:
Work Phone:	Work Phone:
Cell Phone:	Cell Phone:
E-mail:	E-mail:

Name:	Name:
Home Phone:	Home Phone:
Work Phone:	Work Phone:
Cell Phone:	Cell Phone:
E-mail:	E-mail:

Name:	Name:
Home Phone:	Home Phone:
Work Phone:	Work Phone:
Cell Phone:	Cell Phone:
E-mail:	E-mail:

Name:	Name:
Home Phone:	Home Phone:
Work Phone:	Work Phone:
Cell Phone:	Cell Phone:
E-mail:	E-mail:

Name:	Name:
Home Phone:	Home Phone:
Work Phone:	Work Phone:
Cell Phone:	Cell Phone:
E-mail:	E-mail:

Group Contact Information

Name:	Name:
Home Phone:	Home Phone:
Work Phone:	Work Phone:
Cell Phone:	Cell Phone:
E-mail:	E-mail:

Name:	Name:
Home Phone:	Home Phone:
Work Phone:	Work Phone:
Cell Phone:	Cell Phone:
E-mail:	E-mail:

Name:	Name:
Home Phone:	Home Phone:
Work Phone:	Work Phone:
Cell Phone:	Cell Phone:
E-mail:	E-mail:

Name:	Name:
Home Phone:	Home Phone:
Work Phone:	Work Phone:
Cell Phone:	Cell Phone:
E-mail:	E-mail:

Name:	Name:
Home Phone:	Home Phone:
Work Phone:	Work Phone:
Cell Phone:	Cell Phone:
E-mail:	E-mail:

Group Contact Information

Name:		Name:	
Home Phone:		Home Phone:	
Work Phone:		Work Phone:	
Cell Phone:		Cell Phone:	
E-mail:		E-mail:	

Name:		Name:	
Home Phone:		Home Phone:	
Work Phone:		Work Phone:	
Cell Phone:		Cell Phone:	
E-mail:		E-mail:	

Name:		Name:	
Home Phone:		Home Phone:	
Work Phone:		Work Phone:	
Cell Phone:		Cell Phone:	
E-mail:		E-mail:	

Name:		Name:	
Home Phone:		Home Phone:	
Work Phone:		Work Phone:	
Cell Phone:		Cell Phone:	
E-mail:		E-mail:	

Name:		Name:	
Home Phone:		Home Phone:	
Work Phone:		Work Phone:	
Cell Phone:		Cell Phone:	
E-mail:		E-mail:	

Group Prayer Request Record

Date	Name	Request	Answer	Date

Group Prayer Request Record

Date	Name	Request	Answer	Date

Group Prayer Request Record

Date	Name	Request	Answer	Date

Group Prayer Request Record

Date	Name	Request	Answer	Date

Group Prayer Request Record

Date	Name	Request	Answer	Date

Group Prayer Request Record

Date	Name	Request	Answer	Date

CPSIA information can be obtained
at www.ICGtesting.com
Printed in the USA
LVOW04s2325310517
536527LV00006B/575/P

9 780982 034118